INTRODUCTION

Diverticulitis is a common digestive disorder that affects the colon, also known as the large intestine. It occurs when small pouches called diverticula, which can form in the colon's weak areas, become inflamed or infected. When not inflamed, these pouches are usually harmless and result from pressure exerted on the colon over time. However, when they become infected, they can lead to discomfort, pain, and serious complications. Diverticulitis is often associated with a low-fiber diet, which can contribute to the development of these pouches and exacerbate symptoms.

Diverticula themselves are standard, especially as people age. The condition where these pouches become inflamed or infected, known as diverticulitis, presents a range of symptoms. These can include abdominal pain, particularly on the left side, along with bloating, fever, and changes in bowel habits. In severe cases, diverticulitis can lead to complications such as abscesses, perforations, or fistulas, necessitating medical intervention.

Diet plays a crucial role in both the prevention and management of diverticulitis. A low-fiber diet, typically high in refined and processed foods, is considered a significant risk factor. Such a diet can lead to constipation and increased pressure within the colon, potentially causing diverticula to form and become inflamed.

On the other hand, a diverticulitis diet, especially during the acute phase, often begins with clear liquids to provide the colon with rest and relief. A low-fiber diet is usually recommended to reduce irritation as the condition improves. Eventually, transitioning to a high-fiber diet is advised to prevent future episodes and maintain digestive health. Fiber helps soften the stool, preventing constipation and reducing pressure in the colon.

Navigating the diverticulitis diet involves a careful balance of foods that are gentle on the digestive system. This includes incorporating easily digestible items during acute episodes and gradually reintroducing high-fiber foods to promote overall colon health. While the emphasis is on fiber, certain foods, such as nuts, seeds, and popcorn, which can aggravate diverticulitis, are typically limited or avoided.

Understanding diverticulitis and its dietary implications is essential for individuals seeking to manage their symptoms effectively and prevent recurrences. By adopting a balanced diet rich in fiber, staying hydrated, and avoiding specific trigger foods, individuals can take proactive steps to promote digestive wellness and reduce the risk of diverticulitis-related complications. Consulting healthcare professionals and registered dietitians for personalized guidance ensures the most suitable approach to managing this condition, enhancing overall well-being and quality of life.

CHAPTER ONE

Explanation of Diverticula
Formation in the Colon

Diverticula are small, bulging pouches that can form in the lining of the digestive system, particularly in the colon, a part of the large intestine. The process of diverticula formation, known as diverticulosis, is a common occurrence, especially as individuals age. Understanding how these pouches develop sheds light on the complexities of digestive health.

Muscle Weakness and Pressure:

Diverticula usually form in areas of the colon where the muscle layers are naturally weaker. Over time, high pressure within the colon during bowel movements can push the colon's inner lining through these weak spots, creating pouches. The primary cause of this pressure is often a diet low in fiber. A lack of dietary fiber leads to harder stools, requiring increased muscular contractions in the colon to move them, ultimately straining the intestinal walls.

Impact of Low-Fiber Diet:

A low-fiber diet, typical of many Western diets, plays a pivotal role in diverticula formation. Fiber adds bulk to the stool and softens it, making it easier to pass through the colon. When the diet lacks fiber, stools become smaller and more complex, requiring more forceful contractions of the colon muscles during bowel movements. This increased pressure can lead to the formation of diverticula over time.

Aging and Structural Changes:

Aging also contributes to weakening the colon's muscular layers, making older adults more susceptible to diverticulosis. The likelihood of pouch formation increases as the muscles lose their tone and strength. This natural aging process and a low-fiber diet create a conducive environment for diverticula to develop.

Genetic and Lifestyle Factors:

While diet and age are significant factors, genetics may also play a role in diverticula formation. Some individuals may have a genetic predisposition to developing diverticulosis. Additionally, certain lifestyle factors

Complications and Management:

Although diverticula are generally harmless, they can become problematic if inflamed or infected, leading to diverticulitis. To prevent complications, individuals are often advised to adopt a high-fiber diet. A fiber-rich diet promotes regular bowel movements, reduces pressure within the colon, and prevents the formation of hard stools, thereby decreasing the risk of diverticulitis and its associated complications.

CAUSES AND RISK FACTORS OF DIVERTICULITIS

Diverticulitis, the inflammation or infection of small pouches (diverticula) in the colon, can be influenced by various risk factors. Understanding these factors is essential for both prevention and management of this condition. Here are the Causes and Risk Factors of Diverticulitis:

Aging:

Diverticulitis is primarily an age-related condition. The risk increases as people grow older. By the age of 40, many individuals have some diverticula, but the likelihood of inflammation rises significantly in later years.

Low-Fiber Diet:

A diet low in fiber is a significant risk factor for diverticulitis. Fiber adds bulk to stool, softens it, and facilitates easy bowel movements. A lack of fiber results in hard stools, requiring more forceful contractions of the colon muscles during bowel movements. This increased pressure can lead to the formation of diverticula.

Obesity:

Obesity, especially excess abdominal fat, contributes to a higher risk of diverticulitis. Being overweight places additional pressure on the colon, potentially leading to the development of diverticula. Additionally, obesity often correlates with a diet high in processed foods and low in fiber, compounding the risk.

Genetics:

A family history of diverticulitis increases the risk for an individual. If a person's parents or siblings have diverticulitis, they are more likely to develop the condition. Specific genetic factors contributing to this risk are still being studied.

Lifestyle Choices:

Sedentary lifestyles, characterized by a lack of physical activity, are associated with an increased risk of diverticulitis. Regular exercise maintains a healthy weight and promotes overall colon health. Smoking is another detrimental lifestyle choice; it weakens the walls of the colon, making them more prone to diverticula formation.

Certain Medications:

Long-term use of nonsteroidal anti-inflammatory drugs (NSAIDs) like ibuprofen and aspirin can irritate the colon lining, potentially increasing the risk of diverticulitis. Additionally, medications that alter the balance of gut bacteria, such as some antibiotics, might influence diverticulitis risk.

Prior Episodes:

Individuals who have had a previous episode of diverticulitis are more susceptible to recurrent attacks. Each occurrence increases the likelihood of future inflammation, emphasizing the importance of managing the condition effectively through diet and lifestyle modifications.

Connective Tissue Disorders:

Certain connective tissue disorders, such as Ehlers-Danlos syndrome, can weaken the tissues in the colon, making diverticula formation more likely.

Dietary Choices:

Besides low fiber, diets high in red meat and low in fruits and vegetables might elevate the risk of diverticulitis. Red meat, mainly processed varieties, has been associated with a higher incidence of diverticulitis.

SYMPTOMS OF DIVERTICULITIS

Diverticulitis is a condition characterized by the inflammation or infection of small pouches called diverticula, which can develop in the walls of the colon. The symptoms of diverticulitis can vary in intensity, and some individuals may experience mild discomfort while others may face severe complications. Here are the symptoms associated with diverticulitis:

Abdominal Pain:

Abdominal pain, often localized in the lower left side of the abdomen, is a hallmark symptom of diverticulitis. The pain can range from mild cramping to intense, sharp discomfort. In some cases, the pain may become constant and worsen over time.

Changes in Bowel Habits:

Diverticulitis can cause alterations in bowel movements. Some individuals may experience diarrhea, while others may have constipation. Changes in the frequency and consistency of stools are common during diverticulitis episodes.

Fever and Chills:

Inflammation or infection in the diverticula can lead to

systemic symptoms, including fever and chills. Elevated body temperature and shivering are the body's responses to the infection, indicating an immune response.

Nausea and Vomiting:

Individuals with diverticulitis may experience feelings of nausea, sometimes accompanied by vomiting. The inflammation in the digestive tract often triggers these symptoms.

Bloating and Gas:

Increased gas production and bloating can occur due to changes in the gut flora or the accumulation of gas in the inflamed areas. This can lead to discomfort and a feeling of fullness.

Tenderness in the Abdomen:

The affected area of the abdomen may become tender to the touch. Pressing on the abdomen, especially on the lower left side, can cause increased pain or discomfort.

Rectal Bleeding:

In some cases, diverticulitis can cause minor rectal bleeding. This bleeding is usually painless and presents as bright red blood in the stool. However, significant or persistent bleeding requires immediate medical attention.

Urinary Symptoms:

In severe cases, diverticulitis can put pressure on the bladder, leading to urinary symptoms such as increased frequency, urgency, or pain during urination.

Complications:

Complications of diverticulitis can include abscess formation, perforation of the colon, or the development of fistulas (abnormal connections between organs). These complications can cause severe symptoms, including high fever, intense abdominal pain, and sepsis, a life-threatening infection that requires immediate medical intervention.

DIAGNOSIS OF DIVERTICULITIS

Diagnosing diverticulitis involves a careful evaluation of symptoms, physical examinations, and various diagnostic tests to confirm the presence of inflamed or infected diverticula in the colon. A comprehensive approach is essential to ensure accurate diagnosis and appropriate treatment. Here is an overview of the methods used in the diagnosis of diverticulitis:

Medical History and Physical Examination:

A detailed medical history is obtained, focusing on the patient's symptoms, such as abdominal pain, changes in bowel habits, fever, and any history of diverticular disease. During a physical examination, the healthcare provider assesses the abdomen for tenderness, bloating, and signs of infection. The location and intensity of the pain provide valuable clues.

Blood Tests:

Blood tests, including a complete blood count (CBC) and inflammatory markers like C-reactive protein (CRP) and erythrocyte sedimentation rate (ESR), help assess the presence and extent of inflammation in the body. Elevated levels of these markers can suggest an ongoing infection or inflammation, supporting the diagnosis of diverticulitis.

Imaging Studies:

CT Scan (Computed Tomography):

A CT scan of the abdomen and pelvis is the most common imaging test used to diagnose diverticulitis. It provides detailed cross-sectional images of the colon, allowing healthcare providers to identify inflamed diverticula, abscesses, or other complications.

Ultrasound:

Ultrasound imaging can be used to visualize the abdominal area. While less detailed than a CT scan, it can help detect complications such as abscesses or localized inflammation.

Magnetic Resonance Imaging (MRI):

MRI scans can provide detailed images of the abdomen, helping to diagnose diverticulitis and its complications. MRIs are especially useful for patients who cannot undergo CT scans, such as those with allergies to contrast agents.

Colonoscopy:

A colonoscopy may be performed after the acute phase of diverticulitis has resolved to rule out other conditions with similar symptoms, such as inflammatory bowel disease or colorectal cancer. During a colonoscopy, a thin, flexible tube with a camera is inserted into the colon to examine the colon's lining.

Sigmoidoscopy:

Similar to a colonoscopy, a sigmoidoscopy examines the lower part of the colon (sigmoid colon) for signs of diverticulitis. It is less invasive than a colonoscopy and can be helpful in specific cases.

Stool Tests:

Stool tests may be conducted to rule out infections or other gastrointestinal conditions that could be causing symptoms similar to diverticulitis. These tests can identify the presence of blood or signs of infection in the stool.

Barium Enema:

While less common today due to the availability of CT scans, a barium enema involves introducing a contrast material into the colon, making it visible on X-rays. This can help identify diverticula and other abnormalities in the colon.

TREATMENT OF DIVERTICULITIS

Diverticulitis, the inflammation or infection of small pouches in the colon, requires prompt medical attention and appropriate treatment to manage symptoms, prevent complications, and promote healing. The treatment approach varies based on the severity of the condition, the presence of complications, and the individual's overall health. Here are the treatment strategies for diverticulitis:

Dietary Modifications:

During the acute phase of diverticulitis, a clear liquid or low-fiber diet is often recommended to rest the colon and reduce irritation. Clear liquids such as broth, water, and gelatin are easily digestible. As symptoms improve, a gradual transition to a high-fiber diet is encouraged. Fiber softens stools and helps prevent constipation, reducing pressure on the colon. Whole grains, fruits, vegetables, and legumes are excellent sources of dietary fiber.

Antibiotics:

Oral antibiotics are often prescribed to combat the infection and reduce inflammation in cases of mild to moderate diverticulitis without complications. Commonly prescribed antibiotics include ciprofloxacin, metronidazole, or amoxicillin-clavulanate. It's crucial to complete the entire course of antibiotics as defined by the healthcare provider.

Pain Management:

Over-the-counter pain relievers such as acetaminophen may be used to manage pain associated with diverticulitis. Nonsteroidal anti-inflammatory drugs (NSAIDs) like ibuprofen should be avoided, as they can worsen symptoms and irritate the colon.

Hospitalization and Intravenous (IV) Therapy:

Severe cases of diverticulitis, especially those with complications such as abscess formation or significant infection, may require hospitalization. In the hospital, intravenous antibiotics and fluids can be administered to treat the infection and maintain hydration.

Drainage of Abscesses:

If diverticulitis leads to the formation of an abscess (a pus-filled pocket), a procedure may be performed to drain the abscess. This can be done through a needle under imaging guidance or via surgery. Draining the abscess helps alleviate symptoms and prevents the infection from spreading.

Surgery:

Surgery for diverticulitis is usually considered in recurrent, severe, or complicated diverticulitis cases. Surgery may involve removing the affected portion of the colon (colon resection). This procedure can provide relief from recurrent episodes and prevent complications. Laparoscopic (minimally invasive) surgery is often favored due to its quicker recovery times and reduced postoperative pain.

Lifestyle Modifications:

Adopting a healthy lifestyle is essential in managing diverticulitis. Regular physical activity helps maintain a healthy weight and promotes regular bowel movements. Avoiding smoking and excessive alcohol consumption can also support colon health and reduce the risk of recurrent episodes.

Regular Follow-up:

After an episode of diverticulitis, regular follow-up appointments with healthcare providers are crucial. These appointments allow monitoring of the condition, adjustments in treatment if necessary, and discussions about dietary and lifestyle changes to prevent future occurrences.

CHAPTER TWO

Importance of Diet in Managing Diverticulitis Symptoms

Diet plays a pivotal role in managing diverticulitis symptoms, preventing complications, and promoting overall colon health. A well-balanced and fiber-rich diet is particularly crucial for individuals diagnosed with diverticulitis. Here are the importance of diet in managing this condition:

Preventing Symptomatic Flare-ups:

A diet high in fiber, including fruits, vegetables, whole grains, and legumes, helps maintain regular bowel movements. This prevents constipation, which can exacerbate diverticulitis symptoms. Adequate fiber intake softens stools, making them easier to pass and reducing the strain on the colon walls.

Reducing Pressure in the Colon:

High-fiber foods add bulk to stools, allowing them to move more quickly through the colon. This reduces pressure on the colon walls, minimizing the risk of diverticula formation and preventing inflammation of existing diverticula.

Promoting Bowel Regularity:

Fiber-rich foods regulate bowel movements, preventing both diarrhea and constipation. Consistent and regular bowel movements contribute to overall digestive comfort and reduce the risk of diverticulitis episodes.

Encouraging Healthy Gut Microbiota:

A diet rich in fiber nourishes beneficial gut bacteria. These healthy microbes play a vital role in maintaining gut health, supporting the immune system, and reducing inflammation in the colon. A balanced gut microbiota can contribute to preventing and managing diverticulitis symptoms.

Preventing Nutritional Deficiencies:

A well-rounded diet ensures that individuals receive essential nutrients, vitamins, and minerals necessary for overall health. This is particularly important for individuals with diverticulitis, as they may need additional nutrients to support the healing process and boost their immune system.

Minimizing Trigger Foods:

Certain foods, such as nuts, seeds, and popcorn, are traditionally avoided by individuals with diverticulitis due to concerns about these foods getting trapped in the diverticula. A well-planned diet helps individuals identify and avoid trigger foods that may worsen their symptoms or lead to flare-ups.

Supporting Recovery after Flare-ups:

During acute episodes of diverticulitis, a clear liquid or low-fiber diet is often recommended to rest the colon. As symptoms subside, a gradual transition to a high-fiber diet supports the healing process and prevents future episodes.

Promoting Long-term Colon Health:

Adopting a fiber-rich diet is not only essential for

managing diverticulitis symptoms but also for preventing various other colon-related conditions, including colorectal cancer, irritable bowel syndrome (IBS), and inflammatory bowel diseases (IBD). A healthy diet contributes significantly to long-term colon health and overall well-being.

RECOMMENDED FOODS FOR DIVERTICULITIS PATIENTS

A well-balanced diet is crucial for managing diverticulitis symptoms and promoting overall digestive health. When dealing with diverticulitis, it's essential to focus on foods that are gentle on the digestive system, softening the stools and reducing pressure in the colon. Here are the recommended foods for diverticulitis patients:

High-Fiber Foods:

Whole Grains: Opt for whole grains such as brown rice, quinoa, whole wheat pasta, and whole grain bread. These are excellent sources of fiber, promoting regular bowel movements.

Fruits: Include soft, ripe fruits like bananas, applesauce, canned peaches, and ripe melons. Cooked fruits, like stewed apples, can also be easier to digest.

Vegetables: Cooked or steamed vegetables like carrots, spinach, zucchini, and potatoes are gentle on the colon. Well-cooked and peeled vegetables are generally easier to digest.

Lean Proteins:

Chicken and Turkey: Skinless, lean poultry can provide a good source of protein without adding excess fat.

Fish: Fatty fish like salmon, mackerel, and sardines are rich in omega-3 fatty acids, which have anti-inflammatory properties.

Tofu and Tempeh: These plant-based proteins are easy to digest and versatile for various dishes.

Dairy and Alternatives:

Yogurt: Low-fat or non-fat yogurt with probiotics can aid digestion and support a healthy gut.

Lactose-free Milk: For those who are lactose intolerant, lactose-free milk or plant-based milk alternatives like almond, soy, or oat milk can be suitable choices.

Healthy Fats:

Olive Oil: Incorporate olive oil in cooking and salad dressings. It contains monounsaturated fats, which are heart-healthy.

Avocado: Avocados are rich in healthy fats, fiber, and various vitamins. They can be mashed and spread on toast or added to salads.

Fluids:

Water: Staying well-hydrated is essential to prevent constipation. Drink plenty of water throughout the day.

Herbal Teas: Non-caffeinated herbal teas like chamomile or ginger tea can be soothing and aid digestion.

Clear Liquids: During acute flare-ups, clear liquids such as clear broth, water, and plain gelatin can provide necessary hydration without irritating the digestive system.

Avoiding Trigger Foods:

Nuts and Seeds: While these are high in fiber, they are often avoided during acute episodes to prevent irritation.

Popcorn: Popcorn can get stuck in the diverticula, leading to discomfort or inflammation.

Highly Spiced Foods: Spicy foods and excessive use of chili can irritate the colon lining, aggravating symptoms.

Probiotic-Rich Foods:

Yogurt: Besides being a source of protein and calcium, yogurt with live and active cultures can introduce beneficial probiotics into the gut, promoting a healthy balance of bacteria.

Fermented Foods: Sauerkraut, kimchi, and miso are fermented foods rich in probiotics, supporting a healthy gut microbiota.

Moderate Portions and Balanced Meals:

Portion Control: Eating smaller, more frequent meals throughout the day can help manage symptoms and prevent overloading the digestive system.

Balanced Meals: Aim for a balanced combination of fiber, protein, and healthy fats in each meal to promote steady digestion and minimize discomfort.

FOODS TO AVOID AND LIMIT FOR DIVERTICULITIS PATIENTS

Managing diverticulitis involves choosing the right foods and avoiding certain items that can aggravate symptoms or lead to complications. Here are the foods to avoid and limit for diverticulitis patients:

High-Fiber Foods During Flare-ups:

Raw Fruits and Vegetables: While fruits and vegetables are essential, raw ones with skins or seeds can be challenging to digest. Peel and cook them to make them gentler on the digestive system.

Whole Grains: Avoid entire grains like whole wheat bread, bran cereals, and brown rice during flare-ups. These can be rough on the colon. Opt for refined grains temporarily, like white rice and white bread, until symptoms subside.

Beans and Lentils: While they are excellent sources of protein and fiber, beans and lentils can cause gas and bloating. Avoid them or consume them in small amounts, well-cooked and soaked, to reduce gas-producing properties.

High-Fat Foods:

Fried Foods: Fried foods, high in unhealthy fats, can irritate the digestive tract. Avoid fried items like french fries, fried chicken, and chips.

Fatty Cuts of Meat: Fatty meats, especially red meat, can be hard to digest. Opt for lean cuts of poultry and fish instead.

Dairy Products (for lactose intolerant individuals):

Milk and Ice Cream: If lactose intolerant, avoid regular milk and ice cream, as they can cause gas and discomfort. Opt for lactose-free alternatives.

High-Fat Cheese: Cheese, especially high-fat varieties, can be hard to digest. Choose low-fat or small servings of cheese if you tolerate dairy.

Gas-Producing Foods:

Carbonated Drinks: Avoid carbonated beverages, which can lead to bloating and gas.

Cruciferous Vegetables: Vegetables like cabbage, broccoli, and cauliflower are notorious for causing gas. Limit their intake, especially during flare-ups.

Spicy Foods and Irritants:

Spicy Foods: Hot spices and chili can irritate the colon lining. Limit the use of spices, especially during acute episodes.

Caffeine and Alcohol: Both caffeine and alcohol can be dehydrating and irritating to the digestive tract. Limit coffee, tea, and alcohol consumption.

Nuts and Seeds:

Popcorn: The hulls in popcorn can get stuck in the diverticula, leading to inflammation. Avoid popcorn.

Nuts and Seeds: Whole nuts and seeds can be hard to digest. Choose nut butter without added seeds, or opt for finely ground nuts.

Artificial Sweeteners:

Sugar Alcohols: Artificial sweeteners like sorbitol and xylitol, found in sugar-free products, can cause gas and bloating. Read labels and avoid products containing these sweeteners.

Processed Foods:

Processed Meats: Processed meats like sausages, bacon, and deli meats often contain preservatives and high levels of sodium. They can irritate the digestive system. Opt for fresh, unprocessed meats.

Fast Food: Fast food items are often high in unhealthy fats, sodium, and spices. Avoid fast food options as they can trigger symptoms.

Moderation in High-Fructose Foods:

High-Fructose Fruits: Fruits high in fructose, like apples, pears, and watermelon, can cause gas and bloating in some individuals. Consume them in moderation and observe how your body reacts.

Limiting Dairy and Gluten (If Intolerant):

Gluten: For those sensitive to gluten, limiting gluten-containing grains like wheat, barley, and rye can help manage symptoms.

Dairy: If lactose intolerant, choose lactose-free or plant-based dairy alternatives.

SAMPLE MEAL PLAN

Managing diverticulitis through a well-thought-out meal plan is essential for symptom relief and preventing flare-ups. Here are fourteen days meal plans incorporating gentle, easy-to-digest foods to promote colon health:

Day 1:

Breakfast:

• Scrambled Eggs: Soft, scrambled eggs provide protein without irritation.

• White Toast: Refined grains are more accessible to digest during flare-ups.

• Banana: A ripe banana offers potassium and gentle fiber.

Lunch:

• Grilled Chicken Breast: Lean protein helps with muscle repair.

• Mashed Potatoes: Smooth, creamy mashed potatoes are easy on the digestive system.

• Cooked Carrots: Well-cooked carrots provide vitamins and fiber without irritation.

Dinner:

• Baked Salmon: Fatty fish like salmon is rich in omega-3 fatty acids.

• White Rice: Easily digestible, providing energy without

straining the colon.

• Steamed Zucchini: Soft, steamed zucchini is gentle on the stomach.

Snacks:

• Yogurt: Low-fat, probiotic-rich yogurt supports gut health.

• Applesauce: Unsweetened applesauce offers fiber without irritating the skin.

• Rice Cakes: Plain rice cakes are a light, easy-to-digest snack option.

Day 2:

Breakfast:

• Oatmeal: Cooked oats are soft and provide soluble fiber.

• Sliced Peaches: Soft, canned peaches are easy on the stomach.

• Almond Butter: Smooth almond butter on white toast for added protein.

Lunch:

• Turkey Sandwich: Deli turkey breast on white bread, lettuce (without seeds), and mayonnaise.

• Cucumber Salad: Peel and slice cucumbers with a light vinaigrette.

• Ginger Tea: A soothing, anti-inflammatory beverage.

Dinner:

• Baked Chicken Thigh: Moist and tender, providing protein.

• Mashed Sweet Potatoes: Nutrient-rich and more accessible to digest than regular potatoes.

• Steamed Spinach: Soft and packed with vitamins and minerals.

Snacks:

• Yogurt Parfait: Layer yogurt with soft fruits like bananas and add a sprinkle of granola.

• Papaya: Ripe papaya is gentle on the digestive system.

• Rice Pudding: Creamy rice pudding offers a comforting, easy-to-digest dessert.

Day 3:

Breakfast:

• Smoothie: Blend banana, yogurt, almond milk, and a handful of spinach for a nutrient-packed, easy-to-digest breakfast option.

• White Toast: One slice of white toast for added sustenance.

Lunch:

• Tuna Salad: Canned tuna mixed with mayo and served on white bread or crackers.

• Cooked Beets: Soft, cooked beets offer fiber and essential nutrients.

• Ginger Ale: A gentle, non-caffeinated beverage for soothing the stomach.

Dinner:

• Grilled Fish Fillet: Lightly seasoned and grilled for a tender, easy-to-digest main dish.

• White Rice: Accompanied by white rice for a balanced meal.

• Steamed Asparagus: Tender and nutritious, asparagus is

accessible to the digestive system.

Snacks:

• Applesauce with Cinnamon: Unsweetened applesauce with a sprinkle of cinnamon for flavor.

• Rice Cakes with Almond Butter: A satisfying, protein-rich snack option.

• Chamomile Tea: A calming herbal tea to aid digestion and promote relaxation.

Day 4:

Breakfast:

• Greek Yogurt Parfait: Layer Greek yogurt with soft fruits like peaches and top with a sprinkle of granola.

• White Toast: One slice of white toast for added carbohydrates.

• Herbal Tea: Choose a caffeine-free herbal tea for a soothing start to the day.

Lunch:

• Egg Salad Sandwich: Mashed hard-boiled eggs mixed with mayo, served on white bread with lettuce.

• Steamed Green Beans: Tender and easy to digest, providing essential nutrients.

• Coconut Water: A natural, hydrating beverage.

Dinner:

• Roasted Chicken Breast: Seasoned and baked chicken breast for a lean protein source.

• Mashed Butternut Squash: Creamy and rich, butternut squash is gentle on the stomach.

• Boiled Carrots: Soft-boiled carrots offer fiber and vitamins.

Snacks:

• Cottage Cheese: Low-fat cottage cheese is a protein-packed, easy-to-digest snack.

• Melon Slices: Soft melon slices like cantaloupe or honeydew are hydrating and gentle on the stomach.

• Rice Cakes with Jam: Spread a thin layer of fruit jam on rice cakes for a sweet snack.

Day 5:

Breakfast:

• Smoothie Bowl: Blend banana, spinach, and yogurt into a thick consistency. Top with sliced strawberries and a sprinkle of chia seeds.

• White Toast: One slice of white toast for added carbohydrates.

• Decaffeinated Coffee: A mild, decaffeinated coffee for a warm start to the day.

Lunch:

• Salmon Salad: Flaked baked salmon mixed with mayonnaise, served with soft lettuce leaves.

• Cooked Peas: Soft and nutritious, peas are easy on the digestive system.

• Herbal Infusion: Try a calming herbal infusion like chamomile or peppermint tea.

Dinner:

• Tender Beef Stew: Tender chunks of beef cooked with carrots, potatoes, and broth until soft and easy to chew.

• White Rice: Accompanied by white rice for a complete meal.

• Steamed Broccoli: Soft steamed broccoli florets provide fiber and vitamins.

Snacks:

• Applesauce: Unsweetened applesauce is a fiber-rich, easy-to-digest option.

• Pudding Cup: Low-fat pudding cups offer a creamy, soothing dessert.

• Rice Cakes with Nut Butter: Spread a thin layer of nut butter on rice cakes for a protein-rich snack.

Day 6:

Breakfast:

• Porridge: Creamy porridge made with oats and almond milk, topped with sliced bananas, and a drizzle of honey.

• White Toast: One slice of white toast for added carbohydrates.

• Warm Herbal Tea: Choose a warm, herbal tea like ginger or cinnamon for a comforting start.

Lunch:

• Turkey and Cheese Sandwich: Deli turkey breast and low-fat cheese on white bread with lettuce.

• Cooked Spinach: Soft and nutrient-rich, cooked spinach is accessible to the digestive system.

• Decaffeinated Iced Tea: A refreshing, caffeine-free iced tea for hydration.

Dinner:

• Grilled Shrimp: Lightly seasoned and grilled shrimp for a

protein-packed main dish.

• Mashed Potatoes: Creamy mashed potatoes made with a splash of almond milk.

• Boiled Green Beans: Soft-boiled green beans offer fiber and vitamins.

Snacks:

• Yogurt Smoothie: Blend yogurt with ripe berries and a banana for a nutritious and soothing smoothie.

• Peach Slices: Soft, canned peach slices provide vitamins and natural sweetness.

• Rice Cakes with Cottage Cheese: Spread a layer of cottage cheese on rice cakes for a protein-rich snack.

Day 7:

Breakfast:

• Rice Pudding: Creamy rice pudding made with almond milk and a sprinkle of cinnamon.

• Soft Scrambled Eggs: Gently scrambled eggs for added protein.

• Decaffeinated Herbal Tea: A calming herbal tea like lavender or chamomile.

Lunch:

• Tuna Salad Wrap: Canned tuna mixed with mayo, wrapped in a soft tortilla with lettuce and cucumber.

• Boiled Carrots: Soft-boiled carrots are easy to digest and offer nutrients.

• Coconut Water: A natural, hydrating beverage.

Dinner:

• Baked Cod: Baked cod fish with lemon and herbs for a light, protein-rich meal.

• Quinoa: Cooked quinoa for a nutritious, easy-to-digest side dish.

• Steamed Asparagus: Tender asparagus spears are gentle on the digestive system.

Snacks:

• Applesauce with Cinnamon: Unsweetened applesauce with a sprinkle of cinnamon for flavor.

• Cottage Cheese with Pineapple: Low-fat cottage cheese with chunks of canned pineapple for added sweetness.

• Rice Cakes with Almond Butter: A satisfying, protein-rich snack option.

Day 8:

Breakfast:

• Banana Smoothie: Blend banana, almond milk, and a spoonful of almond butter for a creamy, nutrient-packed smoothie.

• White Toast: One slice of white toast for added carbohydrates.

• Decaffeinated Coffee: A mild, decaffeinated coffee for a warm start to the day.

Lunch:

• Egg Drop Soup: Light and soothing egg drop soup with soft-cooked eggs and well-cooked vegetables.

• Steamed Rice: Soft and easily digestible steamed rice as a side.

• Ginger Tea: A calming ginger tea to aid digestion.

Dinner:

• Roasted Chicken Thigh: Moist and tender roasted chicken thigh for a flavorful protein source.

• Mashed Sweet Potatoes: Creamy mashed sweet potatoes with a touch of cinnamon.

• Boiled Green Beans: Soft-boiled green beans provide fiber and nutrients.

Snacks:

• Yogurt with Berries: Low-fat yogurt with soft berries like blueberries or raspberries for added fiber and antioxidants.

• Papaya Smoothie: Blend ripe papaya with yogurt and a drizzle of honey for a soothing and nutritious drink.

• Rice Cakes with Hummus: Spread a thin layer of hummus on rice cakes for a satisfying and protein-rich snack.

Day 9:

Breakfast:

• Rice Porridge: Soft rice porridge made with almond milk and topped with sliced bananas.

• White Toast: One slice of white toast for added carbohydrates.

• Warm Herbal Tea: Choose a warm, herbal tea like peppermint or fennel for a comforting start.

Lunch:

• Grilled Turkey Breast: Grilled turkey breast slices for a lean, protein-packed meal.

• Cooked Carrots and Peas: Soft-cooked carrots and peas for added fiber and nutrients.

• Decaffeinated Iced Tea: A refreshing, caffeine-free iced tea for hydration.

Dinner:

• Baked Salmon: Baked salmon fillet with lemon and dill for a light and nutritious dinner option.

• Quinoa Salad: Quinoa mixed with cooked, soft vegetables like bell peppers and cucumber, dressed with a light vinaigrette.

• Steamed Broccoli: Tender steamed broccoli florets provide fiber and vitamins.

Snacks:

• Yogurt with Soft Granola: Low-fat yogurt with soft granola clusters for added crunch and nutrition.

• Melon Balls: Soft melon balls like cantaloupe or honeydew for a hydrating and gentle snack.

• Rice Cakes with Cottage Cheese: Spread a layer of cottage cheese on rice cakes for a protein-rich and satisfying snack.

Day 10:

Breakfast:

• Yogurt Parfait: Layer low-fat yogurt with ripe strawberries and a sprinkle of granola for added texture.

• White Toast: One slice of white toast for a light breakfast.

• Decaffeinated Herbal Tea: Choose a gentle herbal tea like chamomile or lemon balm.

Lunch:

• Turkey and Avocado Wrap: Deli turkey breast, sliced avocado, and lettuce wrapped in a soft tortilla.

• Boiled Potatoes: Soft-boiled potatoes seasoned with a touch of olive oil and herbs.

• Ginger Infused Water: Add slices of fresh ginger to water for a refreshing beverage.

Dinner:

• Grilled Chicken Tenders: Tender grilled chicken tenders marinated in lemon and herbs.

• Quinoa Salad: Quinoa mixed with diced cucumber, tomatoes, and a light vinaigrette.

• Steamed Carrots: Soft steamed carrots for added fiber and nutrients.

Snacks:

• Applesauce: Unsweetened applesauce is easy to digest and provides natural sweetness.

• Rice Cakes with Nut Butter: Spread almond or peanut butter on rice cakes for a protein-packed snack.

• Melon Smoothie: Blend ripe melon with yogurt and ice for a refreshing and hydrating smoothie.

Day 11:

Breakfast:

• Smoothie Bowl: Blend banana, spinach, and almond milk until smooth. Top with sliced kiwi and a sprinkle of chia seeds.

• White Toast: One slice of white toast for additional carbohydrates.

• Warm Herbal Tea: Choose a warm, calming herbal tea like lavender or mint.

Lunch:

• Egg Salad Sandwich: Mashed hard-boiled eggs mixed with a light mayo, served on white bread with lettuce.

• Steamed Green Beans: Tender steamed green beans for added fiber and vitamins.

• Decaffeinated Iced Tea: A refreshing, caffeine-free iced tea for hydration.

Dinner:

• Baked Cod: Baked cod fish with a squeeze of lemon for a simple and light protein option.

• Mashed Butternut Squash: Creamy mashed butternut squash seasoned with a hint of nutmeg.

• Boiled Asparagus: Soft-boiled asparagus spears provide fiber and nutrients.

Snacks:

• Cottage Cheese: Low-fat cottage cheese is protein-rich and easy to digest.

• Peach Slices: Soft, canned peach slices for a naturally sweet snack.

• Rice Cakes with Hummus: Spread a thin layer of hummus on rice cakes for a satisfying and protein-packed snack.

Day 12:

Breakfast:

• Rice Porridge: Soft rice porridge made with almond milk and sliced strawberries for added flavor.

• White Toast: One slice of white toast for additional carbohydrates.

• Decaffeinated Coffee: A mild, decaffeinated coffee for a warm start to the day.

Lunch:

• Chicken and Rice Soup: Light chicken and rice soup with

well-cooked vegetables and tender chicken pieces.

• Mashed Potatoes: Creamy mashed potatoes provide comfort and easy digestion.

• Herbal Infusion: Choose a calming herbal infusion like chamomile or ginger for a soothing beverage.

Dinner:

• Grilled Shrimp Skewers: Grilled shrimp seasoned with herbs and lemon for a flavorful protein option.

• Quinoa Pilaf: Quinoa mixed with cooked, soft vegetables like bell peppers and onions.

• Steamed Broccoli: Tender steamed broccoli florets for added fiber and nutrients.

Snacks:

• Yogurt Smoothie: Blend yogurt with ripe mango and a handful of spinach for a nutrient-packed and refreshing smoothie.

• Rice Cakes with Cottage Cheese: Spread a layer of low-fat cottage cheese on rice cakes for a protein-rich snack.

• Apple Sauce: Unsweetened apple sauce is easy to digest and offers natural sweetness.

Day 13:

Breakfast:

• Greek Yogurt Bowl: Greek yogurt topped with sliced bananas, soft berries, and a sprinkle of ground flaxseeds for added fiber.

• White Toast: One slice of white toast for a light source of carbohydrates.

• Decaffeinated Herbal Tea: Choose a soothing herbal tea

like lavender or chamomile.

Lunch:

• Salmon Salad: Flaked baked salmon mixed with diced cucumber and avocado, dressed with a light lemon vinaigrette.

• Boiled Potatoes: Soft-boiled potatoes with a sprinkle of fresh dill for flavor.

• Decaffeinated Iced Tea: A refreshing, caffeine-free iced tea for hydration.

Dinner:

• Tender Beef Stir-Fry: Strips of tender beef stir-fried with soft vegetables like bell peppers, zucchini, and carrots.

• Steamed Jasmine Rice: Fragrant and soft jasmine rice to complement the stir-fry.

• Steamed Spinach: Tender cooked spinach leaves for added nutrients.

Snacks:

• Cottage Cheese with Pineapple: Low-fat cottage cheese mixed with chunks of canned pineapple for a sweet and protein-rich snack.

• Rice Cakes with Almond Butter: Spread a thin layer of almond butter on rice cakes for a satisfying and protein-packed snack.

• Melon Balls: Soft melon balls like cantaloupe or honeydew for a hydrating and gentle snack.

Day 14:

Breakfast:

• Smoothie Bowl: Blend banana, spinach, frozen berries,

and almond milk into a thick smoothie. Top with granola and sliced kiwi.

• White Toast: One slice of white toast for additional carbohydrates.

• Warm Herbal Tea: Choose a calming herbal tea like ginger or cinnamon for a comforting start.

Lunch:

• Turkey and Avocado Salad: Sliced deli turkey breast, avocado slices, and mixed greens tossed in a light olive oil and lemon dressing.

• Boiled Eggs: Soft-boiled eggs for added protein.

• Ginger Infused Water: Add slices of fresh ginger to water for a refreshing beverage.

Dinner:

• Grilled Chicken Breast: Tender grilled chicken breast seasoned with herbs and lemon.

• Quinoa Pilaf: Quinoa mixed with sautéed soft vegetables like bell peppers and onions.

• Boiled Carrots: Soft-boiled carrots for added fiber and nutrients.

Snacks:

• Pudding Cup: Low-fat pudding cups for a creamy and satisfying dessert.

• Rice Cakes with Hummus: Spread a thin layer of hummus on rice cakes for a protein-rich and filling snack.

• Peach Slices: Soft, canned peach slices for a naturally sweet snack.

SAMPLE SHOPPING LIST

Creating a diverticulitis-friendly diet starts with mindful grocery shopping. Here is a shopping list tailored for individuals managing diverticulitis, focusing on gentle, easily digestible, and fiber-rich options:

Fruits:

• Bananas: Soft and easily digestible.

• Canned Peaches: Packed in their juice without added sugar.

• Applesauce: Unsweetened and smooth for added fiber.

• Papayas: Ripe papayas are gentle on the stomach.

• Berries: Soft berries like strawberries and blueberries are rich in antioxidants and fiber.

Vegetables:

• Carrots: Soft and versatile, rich in fiber.

• Zucchini: Easy to cook and digest.

• Spinach: Cooked spinach is soft and nutrient-dense.

• Cucumber: Peel and slice it for salads or snacking.

• Bell Peppers: Soft and colorful addition to meals.

• Sweet Potatoes: A nutritious and easily digestible

alternative to regular potatoes.

Grains:

• White Rice: Easily digestible and versatile.

• Quinoa: A protein-rich alternative to traditional grains.

• Oats: Perfect for making porridge or oatmeal.

• White Bread: Refined, soft bread for sandwiches or toasting.

• Rice Cakes: Light and crunchy snack option.

Proteins:

• Chicken Breast: Lean and versatile protein source.

• Turkey: Low-fat deli turkey for sandwiches or salads.

• Fish: Cod, salmon, and other soft-fleshed fish are easy to digest.

• Eggs: Soft-boiled or scrambled eggs provide protein.

• Tofu: Soft and versatile plant-based protein option.

Dairy and Alternatives:

• Low-Fat Yogurt: Probiotic-rich and easy on the stomach.

• Almond Milk: A lactose-free alternative for cooking and drinking.

• Cottage Cheese: Low-fat and protein-packed.

Snacks:

• Almond Butter: Smooth almond butter for spreading on rice cakes or toast.

• Hummus: A fiber and protein-rich dip for veggies or rice cakes.

• Low-Fat Pudding Cups: Creamy and gentle dessert option.

• Herbal Teas: Chamomile, ginger, or peppermint tea for soothing digestion.

• Ginger Ale: A non-caffeinated option to ease stomach discomfort.

Other Essentials:

• Olive Oil: For cooking and salad dressings.

• Honey: Natural sweetener for adding flavor.

• Herbs and Spices: For seasoning, mild options like parsley, dill, and basil.

• Ground Flaxseeds: Rich in fiber, add to yogurt or smoothies.

• Nuts and Seeds (in moderation): Soft varieties like almond and pumpkin seeds.

Supplements (Consult a healthcare provider):

• Probiotics: To promote healthy gut flora.

• Fiber Supplements: If recommended by a healthcare provider to regulate bowel movements.

CHAPTER THREE

Diverticulitis Diet Recipes Guidelines:
Clear Fruit Juice

Meal Description: This Clear Fruit Juice is a light, refreshing beverage made from freshly strained oranges, grapes, and melons. Packed with natural sweetness and vitamins, it's a perfect choice for a healthy and hydrating drink.

Ingredients:

• Two large oranges

• 1 cup red grapes

• 1/2 small melon (such as cantaloupe or honeydew)

Instructions:

1. Preparation:

• Wash all the fruits thoroughly under running water.

• Slice the oranges in half and juice them using a citrus juicer, removing any seeds.

• Destem the grapes and cut the melon, removing seeds and skin. Cut into manageable chunks for juicing.

2. Juicing:

• In a blender, combine the grape chunks and blend until smooth.

• Place a fine mesh sieve or cheesecloth over a clean bowl and gently pour the grape puree over it, pressing to extract the juice. Discard the pulp.

• Repeat the same process with the melon chunks, straining the juice into the bowl.

• Pour the freshly squeezed orange juice into the same bowl.

3. Mixing:

• Stir the three fruit juices together gently to combine them into a harmonious blend.

4. Refrigeration:

• Refrigerate the juice for at least 1-2 hours to chill it thoroughly.

5. Serving:

• Serve the clear fruit juice over ice cubes in glasses.

• Garnish with a slice of orange or a few grapes, if desired.

• Enjoy the refreshing and naturally sweet Clear Fruit Juice immediately.

Nutrition Information (per serving, serves 4):

• Calories: Approximately 150 calories

• Total Fat: 0g

• Cholesterol: 0mg

• Sodium: 2mg

• Total Carbohydrates: 38g

• Dietary Fiber: 2g

• Sugars: 30g

• Protein: 2g

LEMON WATER

Meal Description: Lemon Water is a simple yet refreshing beverage that combines the zesty freshness of freshly squeezed lemon juice with the crispness of ice-cold water. This rejuvenating drink is incredibly refreshing and a delightful way to stay hydrated throughout the day.

Ingredients:

• One fresh lemon

• One glass (about 8 oz) of cold water

• 3-4 ice cubes

• Fresh mint leaves for garnish (optional)

Instructions:

1. Preparation:

• Wash the lemon thoroughly under running water to remove any impurities from the skin.

• Roll the lemon gently on the countertop to soften it, making it easier to juice.

• Prepare a glass of cold water and have the ice cubes ready.

2. Lemon Juice:

• Cut the lemon in half. Squeeze the juice from one-half of the lemon into the glass of cold water. Use a citrus juicer or your hand to extract the juice. Remove any seeds.

3. Ice Cubes:

• Drop 3-4 ice cubes into the glass to make the lemon water refreshing and chilled.

4. Garnish (Optional):

• Garnish your Lemon Water with a few fresh mint leaves for an extra burst of freshness and visual appeal. This step is optional but adds a delightful touch.

5. Stir and Enjoy:

• Stir the lemon water gently with a spoon to mix the lemon juice and chill the water thoroughly.

• Your revitalizing Lemon Water is ready to enjoy!

Nutrition Information (per Serving):

• Calories: Approximately ten calories

• Total Fat: 0g

• Cholesterol: 0mg

• Sodium: 2mg

• Total Carbohydrates: 3g

• Dietary Fiber: 1g

• Sugars: 1g

• Protein: 0g

HOMEMADE VEGETABLE BROTH

Description: This homemade vegetable broth is a nourishing base for soups, stews, and sauces. Made with simple ingredients and a straightforward process, it's delicious and low in calories. Simmering carrots, celery, and onions in water with a pinch of salt creates a clear and flavorful vegetable broth that can enhance the taste of various dishes.

Ingredients:

• Two large carrots, peeled and chopped

• Two celery stalks, chopped

• One large onion, peeled and quartered

• 8 cups water

• Pinch of salt

Instructions:

1. Prepare the Vegetables:

• Peel and chop the carrots into medium-sized chunks.

• Chop the celery stalks into pieces.

• Peel the onion and cut it into quarters.

2. Simmer the Vegetables:

• Combine the chopped carrots, celery, and onions in a large pot.

• Add 8 cups of water to the pot.

• Sprinkle a pinch of salt over the vegetables and water.

3. Bring to a Boil:

• Place the pot on the stove over medium-high heat.

• Bring the mixture to a boil.

4. Simmer:

• Once the broth mixture is boiling, reduce the heat to low to maintain a gentle simmer.

• Let it simmer uncovered for about 1 to 1.5 hours. This allows the flavors to meld and the vegetables to release their essence into the broth.

5. Strain the Broth:

• After simmering, turn off the heat and let the broth cool slightly.

• Carefully strain the broth through a fine mesh sieve or cheesecloth into another pot or large bowl. Press down on the vegetables to extract all the liquid. Discard the solids.

6. Store or Use:

• Your clear and aromatic vegetable broth is ready to use in your favorite recipes.

• If you're not using it immediately, let it cool completely, then store it in airtight containers in the refrigerator for up to 3 days. Alternatively, freeze it for future use.

Nutrition Information (Per Serving, serves 4):

• Calories: Approximately 50 kcal

- Carbohydrates: 12g
- Protein: 2g
- Fat: 0g
- Fiber: 3g
- Sugars: 6g

PEACH OR APRICOT SMOOTHIE

Description: This Peach or Apricot Smoothie is a refreshing and nutritious treat, perfect for a quick breakfast or a healthy snack. This smoothie is delightfully sweet, satisfying, and easy to prepare, made with canned peaches or apricots packed in juice, creamy yogurt, and a handful of ice.

Ingredients:

• 1 cup canned peaches or apricots in juice (not syrup), drained

• 1/2 cup plain or vanilla yogurt

• One handful of ice cubes

Instructions:

1. Prepare the Ingredients:

• Drain the canned peaches or apricots, reserving the juice.

2. Blend the Ingredients:

• Combine the drained peaches or apricots, yogurt, and ice cubes in a blender.

3. Blend Until Smooth:

• Blend the ingredients until smooth and creamy. If the smoothie is too thick, you can add some reserved juice from the canned fruits to reach your desired consistency.

4. Taste and Adjust:

• Taste the smoothie and adjust the sweetness or thickness by adding more fruit or juice if needed.

5. Serve Cold:

• Pour the smoothie into a glass.

• Optionally, garnish with a slice of fresh peach or apricot on the rim of the glass for a decorative touch.

6. Enjoy:

• Grab a straw and immediately enjoy your delicious and refreshing Peach or Apricot Smoothie.

Nutrition Information (Per Serving, serves 1):

• Calories: Approximately 150 kcal

• Carbohydrates: 33g

• Protein: 6g

• Fat: 1g

• Fiber: 2g

• Sugars: 30g

CLEAR FISH BROTH

Description: This Clear Fish Broth is a light and flavorful base for soups, stews, and sauces. Made by simmering fish bones and mild-flavored fish-like soles in water, this clear broth is simple to prepare and serves as an excellent foundation for various seafood dishes.

Ingredients:

• Fish bones (from white fish, such as sole), about 1 pound

• Mild-flavored fish fillets (such as sole or cod), about 1/2 pound

• 8 cups water

• Salt, to taste

Instructions:

1. Prepare the Fish:

• Rinse the fish bones and fillets under cold water to remove impurities.

2. Simmer the Fish:

• Combine the fish bones, mild-flavored fish fillets, and 8 cups of water in a large pot.

3. Bring to a Boil:

• Place the pot on the stove over medium-high heat.

• Bring the mixture to a boil.

4. Reduce Heat and Simmer:

• Once the broth is boiling, reduce the heat to low to maintain a gentle simmer.

• Let it simmer uncovered for about 30-45 minutes. This allows the fish flavors to infuse into the broth.

5. Strain the Broth:

• After simmering, turn off the heat and let the broth cool slightly.

• Carefully strain the broth through a fine mesh sieve or cheesecloth into another pot or large bowl. Press down on the fish solids to extract all the liquid. Discard the solids.

6. Season and Serve:

• Taste the broth and add salt if necessary, depending on your preference.

• Your clear fish broth is ready to be used in soups, stews, or sauces.

7. Store or Use:

• If not using immediately, let the broth cool completely, then store it in airtight containers in the refrigerator for up to 2 days. For more extended storage, freeze the broth in freezer-safe containers.

Nutrition Information (Per Serving, serves 4):

• Calories: Approximately 20 kcal

• Protein: 4g

• Fat: 0g

• Carbohydrates: 0g

• Fiber: 0g

- Sugars: 0g

SOFT SCRAMBLED EGGS

Description: Soft Scrambled Eggs are the epitome of breakfast comfort. This simple yet luxurious dish is made by gently scrambling eggs in a non-stick pan until they are soft, creamy, and velvety. Perfect for a leisurely breakfast or brunch, these eggs practically melt in your mouth.

Ingredients:

• Three large eggs

• Salt, to taste

• Black pepper, freshly ground, to taste

• Two tablespoons butter

• Optional toppings: chopped chives, grated cheese, or diced tomatoes

Instructions:

1. Crack and Whisk the Eggs:

• Crack the eggs into a bowl. Add a pinch of salt and a grind of black pepper. Whisk the eggs gently with a fork or a whisk until the yolks and whites are thoroughly combined.

2. Heat the Pan:

• Place a non-stick pan over low to medium-low heat. Add the butter and let it melt, ensuring it doesn't brown.

3. Scramble the Eggs:

• Pour the whisked eggs into the pan. Let them sit for a few moments without stirring to allow the bottom to set slightly.

4. Gently Stir:

• Using a spatula, gently stir the eggs from the edges to the center. Continue stirring occasionally, allowing the uncooked eggs to come into contact with the pan.

5. Cook to Desired Consistency:

• Continue to cook and gently stir until the eggs are softly set but still slightly runny. Remember, the eggs will continue to cook even after you remove them from the heat due to residual heat in the pan.

6. Remove from Heat:

• Remove the pan from the heat as soon as the eggs reach your desired consistency (they should be creamy and slightly runny). The eggs will continue to cook for a short while off the heat.

7. Serve Immediately:

• Spoon the soft scrambled eggs onto a plate immediately. Garnish with optional toppings like chopped chives, grated cheese, or diced tomatoes, if desired.

8. Enjoy:

• Enjoy your soft scrambled eggs with toast, a bagel, or simply on your own for a decadent and comforting breakfast experience.

Nutrition Information (Per Serving, serves 1):

• Calories: Approximately 210 kcal

- Protein: 18g
- Fat: 15g
- Carbohydrates: 1g
- Fiber: 0g
- Sugars: 0g

PEANUT BUTTER BANANA SMOOTHIE

Description: This Peanut Butter Banana Smoothie is a creamy and indulgent treat that combines the natural sweetness of ripe bananas with the rich taste of peanut butter. Blended with low-fat milk and a touch of honey, this protein-rich smoothie is not only delicious but also a great source of energy.

Ingredients:

• Two ripe bananas, peeled and sliced

• Two tablespoons peanut butter (unsweetened and natural)

• 1 cup low-fat milk (or almond milk for a dairy-free option)

• 1-2 tablespoons honey (or to taste)

• One handful of ice cubes (optional)

• Optional garnish: a sprinkle of cinnamon or a few slices of banana

Instructions:

1. Prepare the Ingredients:

• Peel and slice the ripe bananas.

2. Blend the Ingredients:

• Combine the sliced bananas, peanut butter, low-fat milk,

and honey in a blender.

3. Blend Until Smooth:

• Blend the ingredients on high speed until the mixture is smooth and creamy. If you prefer a thicker smoothie, you can add a handful of ice cubes and blend again until well incorporated.

4. Taste and Adjust:

• Taste the smoothie and adjust the sweetness by adding more honey if necessary. Blend again to combine.

5. Serve Cold:

• Pour the smoothie into glasses.

• Optionally, garnish with a sprinkle of cinnamon or a few slices of banana on top for a decorative touch.

6. Enjoy:

• Insert a straw and immediately enjoy your Peanut Butter Banana Smoothie as a satisfying breakfast, snack, or post-workout refreshment.

Nutrition Information (Per Serving, serves 2):

• Calories: Approximately 250 kcal

• Protein: 9g

• Fat: 11g

• Carbohydrates: 32g

• Fiber: 3g

• Sugars: 19g

YOGURT PARFAIT

Description: A Yogurt Parfait is a delightful and healthy dessert or breakfast option. This recipe layers low-fat yogurt with mashed berries and granola granola (without nuts) to create a delicious and visually appealing treat. It's pleasing to the eye and perfectly balances creamy, fruity, and crunchy textures.

Ingredients:

• 1 cup low-fat yogurt (plain or flavored, as per preference)

• 1 cup mixed berries (such as strawberries, blueberries, raspberries), mashed

• 1/2 cup GranolaGranola (without nuts)

• 1-2 tablespoons honey or maple syrup (optional for sweetness)

• Fresh mint leaves for garnish (optional)

Instructions:

1. Prepare the Berries:

• Wash and mash the mixed berries with a fork or a potato masher until they form a chunky puree. You can blend the berries in a blender if you prefer a smoother texture.

2. Assemble the Parfait:

• Start by layering about 1/4 cup of low-fat yogurt at the bottom in a glass or a bowl.

3. Add Mashed Berries:

• Add a layer of the mashed berries on top of the yogurt, using about 1/4 cup of the berry puree.

4. Sprinkle GranolaGranola:

• Sprinkle two tablespoons of granola granola (without nuts) over the berry layer. This provides a crunchy texture to the parfait.

5. Repeat the Layers:

• Repeat the layers with another 1/4 cup of yogurt, 1/4 cup of mashed berries, and two tablespoons of granola granola until the glass or bowl is filled, ending with a layer of granola granola on top.

6. Drizzle with Honey (Optional):

• If you prefer extra sweetness, drizzle 1-2 tablespoons of honey or maple syrup over the top layer.

7. Garnish (Optional):

• Garnish the parfait with fresh mint leaves for a burst of color and added freshness.

8. Serve Immediately or Refrigerate:

• Serve the Yogurt Parfait immediately as a delicious, healthy dessert or breakfast option. Alternatively, cover and refrigerate for later consumption.

Nutrition Information (Per Serving, serves 1):

• Calories: Approximately 300 kcal

• Protein: 12g

• Fat: 6g

• Carbohydrates: 55g

- Fiber: 6g
- Sugars: 26g

TENDER TURKEY MEATBALLS

Description: These Tender Turkey Meatballs are a healthier alternative to traditional meatballs, made with lean ground turkey, breadcrumbs, egg, and flavorful seasonings. Baked to perfection, these meatballs are tender, moist, and packed with delicious flavors. They are versatile and can be served with pasta, in sandwiches, or as appetizers.

Ingredients:

• 1 pound lean ground turkey

• 1/2 cup breadcrumbs

• One large egg, lightly beaten

• Two cloves garlic, minced

• 1/4 cup grated Parmesan cheese

• One teaspoon dried oregano

• One teaspoon of dried basil

• 1/2 teaspoon salt

• 1/4 teaspoon black pepper

• 1/4 teaspoon red pepper flakes (optional, for a bit of heat)

• Cooking spray or olive oil for greasing

Instructions:

1. Preheat the Oven:

• Preheat your oven to 375°F (190°C).

2. Prepare the Meatball Mixture:

• In a large mixing bowl, combine the ground turkey, breadcrumbs, beaten egg, minced garlic, grated Parmesan cheese, dried oregano, dried basil, salt, black pepper, and red pepper flakes (if using). Mix well until all ingredients are evenly incorporated.

3. Shape the Meatballs:

• Lightly grease your hands with a bit of oil or water to prevent sticking. Roll small portions of the mixture between your palms to form meatballs, about 1 to 1.5 inches in diameter. Place the formed meatballs on a baking sheet lined with parchment paper.

4. Bake the Meatballs:

• Arrange the meatballs on the prepared baking sheet. Bake in the preheated oven for 20-25 minutes or until the meatballs are cooked through and no longer pink in the center. The internal temperature of the meatballs should reach 165°F (74°C).

5. Serve:

• Remove the meatballs from the oven and let them rest for a few minutes before serving. Serve hot with your favorite sauce pasta, or enjoy them as appetizers.

Nutrition Information (Per Serving, makes about 20 meatballs):

• Calories: Approximately 45 kcal per meatball

• Protein: 6g

• Fat: 2g

- Carbohydrates: 3g
- Fiber: 0g
- Sugars: 0g

CLEAR CHICKEN BROTH

Description: Clear Chicken Broth is a light and nourishing base, perfect for soups, sauces, and various culinary creations. Simmered with chicken bones, vegetables, and seasonings, this clear broth is strained to perfection, resulting in a flavorful, golden liquid that's both comforting and versatile.

Ingredients:

- 1 pound chicken bones (such as carcass or wings)

- 8 cups water

- One onion, peeled and quartered

- 2 carrots, washed and cut into chunks

- Two celery stalks, washed and cut into chunks

- Two cloves garlic, peeled and smashed

- One bay leaf

- 4-5 whole black peppercorns

- Salt, to taste

Instructions:

1. Prepare the Ingredients:

- Rinse the chicken bones under cold water to remove

any impurities. Cut the vegetables into chunks for easier handling during cooking.

2. Simmer the Chicken Broth:

• Combine the chicken bones, onion, carrots, celery, garlic, bay leaf, and whole black peppercorns in a large pot. Pour in 8 cups of water.

3. Bring to a Boil:

• Place the pot on the stove over medium-high heat. Bring the mixture to a boil. As the broth comes to a boil, skim off any foam or impurities that rise to the surface using a spoon.

4. Reduce Heat and Simmer:

• Once the broth reaches a rolling boil, reduce the heat to low to maintain a gentle simmer. Cover the pot partially with a lid and let it simmer for about 1.5 to 2 hours. This allows the flavors to meld and the broth to become rich and flavorful.

5. Strain the Broth:

• After simmering, turn off the heat and let the broth cool slightly. Carefully strain the broth through a fine mesh sieve, cheesecloth, or a muslin cloth into another pot or large bowl. Press down on the solids to extract all the liquid. Discard the solids.

6. Season with Salt:

• Taste the broth and season with salt, as needed, to enhance the flavors. Be mindful of the salt, as you can always add more later.

7. Serve or Store:

• Use the clear chicken broth immediately in your favorite

recipes, or store it in airtight containers once cooled. Refrigerate for up to 3-4 days or freeze for a longer shelf life.

Nutrition Information (Per Serving, based on 1 cup):

• Calories: Approximately 20 kcal

• Protein: 2g

• Fat: 0g

• Carbohydrates: 4g

• Fiber: 1g

• Sugars: 2g

VEGETABLE CLEAR SOUP

Description: Vegetable Clear Soup is a light, comforting, and flavorful dish made by boiling a medley of fresh vegetables. This simple yet nutritious soup highlights the natural goodness of vegetables like carrots, zucchini, and celery, creating a transparent and delicate broth. Perfect as an appetizer or a light meal, this soup is a refreshing way to enjoy the essence of fresh vegetables.

Ingredients:

- 4 cups water

- One large carrot, peeled and sliced

- One medium zucchini, sliced

- Two celery stalks, sliced

- Salt and pepper, to taste

- Fresh parsley, chopped, for garnish (optional)

Instructions:

1. Prepare the Vegetables:

- Peel and slice the carrot. Wash and slice the zucchini and celery stalks. Cut the vegetables into uniform, bite-sized pieces.

2. Boil the Vegetables:

• In a pot, bring 4 cups of water to a boil. Add the sliced carrots, zucchini, and celery to the boiling water. Reduce the heat to medium-low and simmer the vegetables until they are tender but still slightly crisp, about 8-10 minutes.

3. Strain the Broth:

• Remove the boiled vegetables from the pot using a fine mesh sieve or a slotted spoon, leaving only the clear broth.

4. Season the Soup:

• Season the clear vegetable broth with salt and pepper to taste. Be mindful of the salt, as the broth should be delicately flavored.

5. Garnish and Serve:

• Ladle the clear vegetable soup into bowls. Garnish with fresh chopped parsley, if desired, for a burst of color and added freshness.

6. Serve Hot:

• Serve the Vegetable Clear Soup hot as an appetizer or a light and nourishing meal. Enjoy the delicate flavors of the fresh vegetables in this clear and comforting soup.

Nutrition Information (Per Serving, serves 4):

• Calories: Approximately 30 kcal

• Protein: 1g

• Fat: 0g

• Carbohydrates: 7g

• Fiber: 2g

• Sugars: 4g

SUGAR-FREE GELATIN CUPS

Description: Sugar-Free Gelatin Cups are a delightful, low-calorie dessert that is easy to make and perfect for satisfying your sweet cravings. Prepared with sugar-free gelatin, these colorful and refreshing cups are a guilt-free treat. Enjoyed chilled, they make a great dessert for parties, picnics, or as a light, satisfying snack.

Ingredients:

• One package (0.3 oz or 8g) sugar-free flavored gelatin mix (any flavor of your choice)

• 1 cup boiling water

• 1 cup cold water

• Fresh berries or sugar-free whipped topping for garnish (optional)

Instructions:

1. Prepare the Gelatin:

• In a heatproof bowl, dissolve the sugar-free flavored gelatin mix in 1 cup of boiling water. Stir until completely dissolved.

2. Add Cold Water:

• Add 1 cup of cold water to the dissolved gelatin mixture.

Stir well to combine.

3. Pour into Cups:

• Carefully pour the gelatin mixture into cups or small dessert glasses, dividing it evenly among them.

4. Refrigerate Until Set:

• Place the cups in the refrigerator and let the gelatin set. This usually takes about 2-4 hours, but follow the package instructions for specific setting times.

5. Garnish (Optional):

• Before serving, you can garnish the gelatin cups with fresh berries or a dollop of sugar-free whipped topping for an extra touch of flavor and presentation.

6. Serve Cold:

• Once the gelatin is fully set, remove the cups from the refrigerator. Serve the sugar-free gelatin cups chilled, and enjoy this guilt-free, sweet treat.

Nutrition Information (Per Serving, makes 4 cups):

• Calories: Approximately 10 kcal

• Protein: 1g

• Fat: 0g

• Carbohydrates: 0g

• Fiber: 0g

• Sugars: 0g

FRUIT JUICE POPSICLES

Description: Fruit Juice Popsicles are a refreshing and wholesome treat, especially during hot weather. Made with your favorite fruits, a touch of honey, and water, these homemade popsicles are delicious and free from artificial flavors and sugars. Enjoy the natural sweetness and vibrant flavors of your favorite fruits in frozen form!

Ingredients:

• 2 cups fresh fruits (such as strawberries, mangoes, pineapples, or a mix of your choice), peeled, pitted, and chopped

• 1/4 cup water

• 1-2 tablespoons honey or agave syrup (optional, depending on the sweetness of your fruits)

Instructions:

1. Prepare the Fruits:

• Peel, pit, and chop the fresh fruits into small chunks, removing any seeds or pits.

2. Blend the Fruits:

• In a blender, combine the chopped fruits, water, and honey (if using). Blend until smooth and well combined. Taste the mixture and adjust the sweetness by adding more honey if needed.

3. Pour into Popsicle Molds:

• Carefully pour the blended fruit mixture into popsicle molds, leaving a little space at the top for expansion during freezing. Insert popsicle sticks into the center of each mold.

4. Freeze the Popsicles:

• Place the popsicle molds in the freezer and let them freeze for at least 4-6 hours or until completely solid. For best results, freeze them overnight.

5. Unmold and Enjoy:

• To unmold the popsicles, run the molds briefly under warm water to loosen the popsicles. Gently pull the popsicles out of the molds and enjoy your homemade Fruit Juice Popsicles immediately!

6. Optional: Customize Your Popsicles:

• Feel free to get creative and customize your popsicles by adding slices of fresh fruits, berries, or even mint leaves into the molds before pouring the fruit mixture. This adds visual appeal and extra freshness to your popsicles.

7. Serve and Stay Refreshed:

• Serve these naturally sweet and fruity popsicles to beat the heat on a sunny day. They're perfect for kids and adults alike, offering a burst of natural flavors and a refreshing way to enjoy your favorite fruits.

HERBAL LEMON TEA

Description: Herbal Lemon Tea is a soothing and refreshing beverage made by steeping chamomile or mint tea bags in hot water and enhancing the flavor with a slice of lemon. This delightful tea offers the calming benefits of chamomile or the refreshing taste of mint, combined with the bright citrus notes from lemon. It's a perfect way to unwind and enjoy a moment of relaxation.

Ingredients:

• One chamomile or mint tea bag

• 1 cup hot water

• One slice of lemon

• Optional: honey or your preferred sweetener to taste

Instructions:

1. Boil Water:

• Boil 1 cup of water in a kettle or on the stovetop until it reaches the desired temperature for steeping your tea.

2. Steep the Tea Bag:

• Place the chamomile or mint tea bag in a cup. Pour the hot water over the tea bag.

3. Steeping Time:

• Let the tea bag steep in hot water for 3-5 minutes, or follow the package instructions for the recommended steeping time. Longer steeping can result in a more robust flavor, but be cautious not to over-steep, as it can make the tea bitter.

4. Add Lemon Slice:

• After steeping, remove the tea bag and add a slice of lemon to the tea. The lemon adds a refreshing citrus flavor that complements the herbal notes of the tea.

5. Optional: Sweeten to Taste:

• Add honey or sweetener to the tea if you prefer a sweeter taste. Stir until the sweetener is completely dissolved. Taste and adjust the sweetness according to your preference.

6. Enjoy:

• Stir the tea gently, allowing the lemon slice to infuse its flavor. Take a moment to inhale the soothing aroma and then savor your Herbal Lemon Tea. Enjoy it hot and freshly brewed.

CREAMY CARROT SOUP

Description: Creamy Carrot Soup is a velvety and comforting dish showcasing carrots' natural sweetness. Boiled until soft and then blended with low-fat milk, this soup is not only delicious but also healthy and satisfying. Seasoned with a touch of salt and pepper, this soup is a perfect choice for a warm, nourishing meal.

Ingredients:

• 1 pound (about 450g) carrots, peeled and sliced

• 4 cups water or vegetable broth

• 1 cup low-fat milk

• Salt and pepper, to taste

• Fresh parsley, chopped, for garnish (optional)

• Croutons or a dollop of low-fat yogurt for garnish (optional)

Instructions:

1. Boil the Carrots:

• Combine the sliced carrots and water (or vegetable broth) in a large pot. Bring to a boil over medium-high heat. Reduce the heat to low, cover the pot, and simmer until the carrots are very soft, about 20-25 minutes.

2. Blend the Carrots:

• Using a blender or an immersion blender, carefully blend the cooked carrots with low-fat milk until smooth and creamy. Be cautious when blending hot liquids to avoid splattering. Blend in batches if necessary.

3. Season with Salt and Pepper:

• Return the blended soup to the pot. Season with salt and pepper to taste. Stir well to combine, adjusting the seasoning as needed.

4. Heat and Serve:

• Gently reheat the soup over low heat if necessary. Be careful not to boil the soup once the milk has been added to prevent curdling.

5. Garnish and Serve:

• Ladle the creamy carrot soup into bowls. Garnish with chopped fresh parsley, croutons, or a dollop of low-fat yogurt, if desired, for added texture and flavor.

6. Enjoy:

• Serve the Creamy Carrot Soup hot with a slice of crusty bread or a light salad. Enjoy the rich and comforting flavors of this nutritious soup.

Nutrition Information (Per Serving, serves 4):

• Calories: Approximately 80 kcal

• Protein: 3g

• Fat: 1g

• Carbohydrates: 16g

• Fiber: 4g

• Sugars: 8g

HERB-BAKED CHICKEN BREAST

Description: Herb-Baked Chicken Breast is a simple yet flavorful dish that highlights the natural taste of chicken. Seasoned with aromatic herbs and baked to perfection, this dish results in tender and juicy chicken breasts. This recipe is perfect for a quick and healthy dinner, offering a delicious meal that's easy to prepare.

Ingredients:

• Two boneless, skinless chicken breasts

• Two tablespoons of olive oil

• Two teaspoons of mixed dried herbs (such as thyme, rosemary, and oregano)

• Salt and black pepper, to taste

• Two cloves garlic, minced (optional for added flavor)

• Fresh parsley, chopped, for garnish (optional)

Instructions:

1. Preheat the Oven:

• Preheat your oven to 375°F (190°C).

2. Prepare the Chicken Breast:

• Pat the chicken breasts dry with paper towels. This helps the herbs adhere to the chicken better. If the breasts are thick, you can butterfly them to ensure even cooking.

3. Season the Chicken:

• Mix the olive oil, dried herbs, salt, black pepper, and minced garlic (if used). Brush the herb mixture evenly over both sides of the chicken breasts, ensuring they are well coated.

4. Bake the Chicken:

• Place the seasoned chicken breasts on a baking sheet lined with parchment paper or a silicone baking mat. Bake in the preheated oven for 20-25 minutes or until the chicken is cooked through and reaches an internal temperature of 165°F (74°C). Cooking time may vary based on the thickness of the chicken breasts.

5. Rest and Garnish:

• Remove the chicken from the oven and let it rest for a few minutes. This redistributes the juices, ensuring a juicy and tender result. Garnish with fresh chopped parsley, if desired, for a pop of color and added freshness.

6. Serve:

• Slice the herb-baked chicken breast and serve immediately. Pair it with your favorite vegetables, salad, or grains for a complete and satisfying meal.

Nutrition Information (Per Serving, serves 2):

• Calories: Approximately 250 kcal

• Protein: 26g

• Fat: 15g

• Carbohydrates: 1g

• Fiber: 0g

- Sugars: 0g

PASTA WITH BUTTER AND HERBS

Description: Pasta with Butter and Herbs is a classic and simple dish that emphasizes the natural flavors of pasta, enhanced with the richness of butter and the aromatic touch of herbs. This quick and easy recipe results in a satisfying meal that's perfect for busy weeknights. Delight in the subtle richness of butter, the savory notes of herbs, and the comforting texture of perfectly cooked pasta.

Ingredients:

• 8 ounces (225g) soft pasta (such as linguine, fettuccine, or spaghetti)

• Two tablespoons unsalted butter

• 1-2 tablespoons olive oil

• Two cloves garlic, minced

• One teaspoon mixed dried herbs (such as basil, parsley, and thyme)

• Salt and black pepper, to taste

• Grated Parmesan cheese for serving (optional)

• Fresh basil leaves, chopped, for garnish (optional)

Instructions:

1. Cook the Pasta:

• Cook the soft pasta according to the package instructions in a large pot of salted boiling water until al dente. Drain the pasta, reserving a small amount of pasta water, and set aside.

2. Prepare the Butter Sauce:

• Melt the unsalted butter and olive oil in a large skillet over medium heat. Add the minced garlic and sauté until fragrant, about 1-2 minutes, being careful not to brown the garlic.

3. Toss with Pasta:

• Add the cooked and drained pasta to the skillet. Toss well to coat the pasta evenly with the butter and garlic mixture.

4. Add Herbs:

• Sprinkle the mixed dried herbs over the pasta. Toss again to incorporate the herbs into the dish. Season with salt and black pepper to taste. If the pasta seems dry, you can add a splash of the reserved pasta water to create a silky sauce.

5. Garnish and Serve:

• Transfer the pasta to serving plates. Garnish with grated Parmesan cheese and freshly chopped basil leaves, if desired, for added flavor and presentation.

6. Enjoy:

• Serve the Pasta with Butter and Herbs immediately, savoring the simplicity of this comforting dish. Enjoy the delicate balance of buttery richness and herb-infused pasta goodness.

Nutrition Information (Per Serving, serves 2):

• Calories: Approximately 400 kcal

• Protein: 8g

- Fat: 18g
- Carbohydrates: 52g
- Fiber: 2g
- Sugars: 1g

HOMEMADE APPLESAUCE WITH CINNAMON

Description: Homemade Applesauce with Cinnamon is a delightful and healthy treat made from fresh apples, enhanced with Cinnamon's warm and comforting flavor. This simple recipe transforms soft-boiled apples into a smooth, naturally sweet applesauce with a hint of spice. Enjoy it as a snack, dessert, or a versatile ingredient in various recipes.

Ingredients:

• 4-5 medium-sized apples (such as Gala, Fuji, or Honeycrisp), peeled, cored, and chopped

• 1/4 cup water

• 1/2 teaspoon ground cinnamon (adjust to taste)

• 1-2 tablespoons honey or maple syrup (optional, depending on sweetness preference)

Instructions:

1. Prepare the Apples:

• Peel, core, and chop the apples into small chunks.

2. Boil the Apples:

• In a saucepan, combine the chopped apples and water. Cover and cook over medium heat, stirring occasionally, until the apples are soft and easily mashable. This usually takes about 10-15 minutes.

3. Mash the Apples:

• Once the apples are soft, remove the saucepan from the heat. Use a potato masher or a fork to mash the apples to your desired consistency. You can use a blender or food processor if you prefer a smoother texture.

4. Add Cinnamon:

• Sprinkle ground cinnamon over the mashed apples. Stir well to combine. Adjust the amount of Cinnamon according to your taste preferences.

5. Sweeten (if desired):

• Taste the applesauce. You can add honey or maple syrup if you prefer to be sweeter. Stir until the sweetener is completely incorporated. Note that the sweetness of the apples may vary, so adjust accordingly.

6. Cool and Serve:

• Let the applesauce cool to room temperature. Transfer it to a jar or airtight container and refrigerate until chilled. Homemade applesauce can be served cold or at room temperature.

7. Enjoy:

• Serve the Homemade Applesauce with Cinnamon as a snack, dessert, or accompaniment to various dishes. It's delicious on its own, over yogurt, or as a topping for pancakes and oatmeal.

Nutrition Information (Per Serving, serves 4):

- Calories: Approximately 70 kcal
- Protein: 0g
- Fat: 0g
- Carbohydrates: 18g
- Fiber: 3g
- Sugars: 14g

BAKED LEMON HERB SALMON

Description: Baked Lemon Herb Salmon is a light, flavorful, and healthy dish that brings out the natural taste of salmon. Marinated with zesty lemon juice and aromatic herbs, the salmon fillets are baked to perfection, resulting in a tender and flaky texture. This easy-to-make recipe is perfect for a quick weeknight dinner or a special occasion meal.

Ingredients:

• Two salmon fillets (6-8 ounces each), skin-on or skinless

• Two tablespoons of fresh lemon juice

• Two tablespoons of olive oil

• Two cloves garlic, minced

• One teaspoon of fresh parsley chopped

• 1/2 teaspoon dried dill

• Salt and black pepper, to taste

• Lemon slices, for garnish

• Fresh parsley, chopped, for garnish

Instructions:

1. Preheat the Oven:

• Preheat your oven to 375°F (190°C).

2. Prepare the Salmon:

• Pat the salmon fillets dry with paper towels. If using skin-on salmon, place the fillets skin-side down on a baking sheet lined with parchment paper or aluminum foil.

3. Prepare the Marinade:

• Whisk together the fresh lemon juice, olive oil, minced garlic, chopped parsley, dried dill, salt, and black pepper in a small bowl.

4. Marinate the Salmon:

• Place the salmon fillets in a shallow dish or a resealable plastic bag. Pour the marinade over the salmon, ensuring that each fillet is well coated. Let the salmon marinate for at least 15-20 minutes to absorb the flavors.

5. Bake the Salmon:

• Transfer the marinated salmon fillets to the prepared baking sheet. Bake in the preheated oven for 12-15 minutes or until the salmon is cooked through and flakes easily with a fork. Cooking time may vary based on the thickness of the fillets.

6. Garnish and Serve:

• Remove the baked salmon from the oven. Garnish with lemon slices and freshly chopped parsley for a burst of color and freshness.

7. Enjoy:

• Serve the Baked Lemon Herb Salmon hot with your favorite side dishes, such as steamed vegetables, rice, or a fresh salad. Enjoy the succulent and flavorful salmon with the bright citrus and herb notes.

Nutrition Information (Per Serving, serves 2):

• Calories: Approximately 350 kcal

• Protein: 34g

• Fat: 22g

• Carbohydrates: 2g

• Fiber: 0g

• Sugars: 0g

BROWN RICE BOWL WITH BLACK BEANS, AVOCADO, AND SALSA

Description: Brown Rice Bowl with Black Beans, Avocado, and Salsa is a wholesome and satisfying meal that combines the nutty flavor of brown rice with the protein-rich black beans, creamy avocado slices, and the vibrant freshness of salsa. This bowl is delicious and packed with nutrients, making it a perfect choice for a quick and nutritious lunch or dinner.

Ingredients:

• 1 cup brown rice, cooked according to package instructions

• One can (15 oz) black beans, drained and rinsed

• One ripe avocado, sliced

• 1/2 cup salsa (homemade or store-bought)

• Fresh cilantro leaves, chopped, for garnish

• Lime wedges for serving

• Salt and black pepper, to taste

Instructions:

1. Cook Brown Rice:

• Cook the brown rice according to the package instructions. Fluff the rice with a fork once cooked and set aside.

2. Prepare Black Beans:

• Heat the drained and rinsed black beans in a small saucepan over medium heat until warmed through. Season with a pinch of salt and black pepper. Remove from heat and set aside.

3. Slice Avocado:

• Slice the ripe avocado and sprinkle it with a bit of salt to enhance the flavor.

4. Assemble the Bowl:

• Divide the cooked brown rice among serving bowls. Top with the warmed black beans, avocado slices, and salsa.

5. Garnish and Serve:

• Garnish the brown rice bowl with fresh cilantro leaves. Serve the bowl with lime wedges on the side for an extra burst of citrus flavor.

6. Enjoy:

• Dive into your delicious and nutritious Brown Rice Bowl with Black Beans, Avocado, and Salsa. Mix the ingredients in the bowl to combine the flavors, and squeeze fresh lime juice over the top if desired.

Nutrition Information (Per Serving, serves 2):

• Calories: Approximately 400 kcal

• Protein: 12g

- Fat: 17g
- Carbohydrates: 57g
- Fiber: 13g
- Sugars: 3g

GRILLED MEDITERRANEAN VEGETABLES

Description: Grilled Mediterranean Vegetables are a delightful and healthy side dish that showcases the natural flavors of zucchini, eggplant, and bell peppers. Grilled to perfection, these vegetables are drizzled with olive oil and sprinkled with salt, creating a smoky, savory, and utterly delicious dish. Perfect as a side for grilled meats or as a standalone vegetarian option.

Ingredients:

• Two zucchinis, sliced into rounds

• One eggplant, sliced into rounds or lengthwise

• Two bell peppers (assorted colors) cut into strips

• 2-3 tablespoons olive oil

• Salt, to taste

• Fresh basil leaves, chopped, for garnish (optional)

Instructions:

1. Preheat the Grill:

• Preheat your grill to medium-high heat.

2. Prepare the Vegetables:

• Slice the zucchini, eggplant, and bell peppers according to the specified shapes and sizes.

3. Grill the Vegetables:

• Brush the vegetable slices with olive oil on both sides. Place the vegetables on the grill and cook until they have grill marks and are tender, usually 3-4 minutes per side for zucchini and eggplant and 2-3 minutes per side for bell peppers. Grill times may vary based on your grill's heat intensity.

4. Season with Salt:

• Remove the grilled vegetables from the grill and immediately sprinkle with salt while they are still hot. The salt enhances the natural flavors of the vegetables.

5. Garnish (Optional) and Serve:

• Transfer the grilled vegetables to a serving platter. Garnish with freshly chopped basil leaves, if desired, for a burst of color and added freshness.

6. Enjoy:

• Serve the Grilled Mediterranean Vegetables hot as a side dish, or combine them with pasta, quinoa, or couscous for a wholesome vegetarian meal. Enjoy the smoky and savory flavors of these perfectly grilled vegetables.

Nutrition Information (Per Serving, serves 4):

• Calories: Approximately 120 kcal

• Protein: 2g

• Fat: 7g

• Carbohydrates: 15g

• Fiber: 7g

- Sugars: 8g

FRESH AND ZESTY FRUIT SALAD

Description: Fresh and Zesty Fruit Salad is a vibrant and refreshing combination of diced melons, berries, and kiwi, elevated with a zesty squeeze of lime juice. This colorful fruit salad bursts with natural sweetness and a hint of citrus, making it a delightful and healthy dessert or snack option for any occasion.

Ingredients:

• 1 cup diced watermelon

• 1 cup diced cantaloupe or honeydew melon

• 1 cup fresh strawberries, hulled and halved

• 1 cup blueberries

• Two kiwis, peeled and diced

• Juice of 1-2 limes, to taste

• Fresh mint leaves, for garnish (optional)

Instructions:

1. Prepare the Fruits:

• Wash and dice the watermelon, cantaloupe, strawberries, and kiwis into bite-sized pieces. If using honeydew melon, peel and chop it as well.

2. Combine the Fruits:

• Combine the diced watermelon, cantaloupe, strawberries, blueberries, and kiwis in a large mixing bowl.

3. Add Lime Juice:

• Squeeze the juice of 1-2 limes over the mixed fruits. Start with the juice of one lime and adjust to taste. The lime juice adds a refreshing zing to the fruit salad and enhances the natural flavors.

4. Gently Toss:

• Gently toss the fruits and lime juice together to ensure the fruits are evenly coated with the citrusy goodness.

5. Chill and Garnish:

• Refrigerate the fruit salad for at least 30 minutes to allow the flavors to meld. Before serving, give it a gentle toss again. Optionally, garnish with fresh mint leaves for a pop of color and added freshness.

6. Enjoy:

• Serve the Fresh and Zesty Fruit Salad chilled as a healthy dessert, snack, or a refreshing side dish. It's perfect for summer gatherings or any time you crave a sweet and tangy treat.

Nutrition Information (Per Serving, serves 4):

• Calories: Approximately 80 kcal

• Protein: 1g

• Fat: 0g

• Carbohydrates: 20g

• Fiber: 3g

• Sugars: 14g

CONCLUSION

In conclusion, managing diverticulitis through a well-planned diet is crucial for individuals seeking relief from symptoms and preventing future complications. Diverticulitis, characterized by inflamed or infected pouches in the colon, often finds its roots in a low-fiber diet and poor digestive habits. Understanding the condition and adopting a tailored approach to nutrition can significantly improve the quality of life for those affected.

The journey begins with awareness. Recognizing the symptoms of diverticulitis, such as abdominal pain, bloating, and changes in bowel habits, allows for early intervention. A clear understanding of the diverticulitis diet is equally vital. During acute episodes, clear liquids provide rest to the digestive system, followed by a low-fiber diet to reduce irritation. Gradually, reintroducing high-fiber foods ensures the colon remains healthy, preventing constipation and reducing the risk of diverticula becoming inflamed.

Crucially, individuals must be mindful of what they consume. Avoiding trigger foods like nuts, seeds, and popcorn, which can aggravate diverticulitis, is pivotal.

Instead, embracing a diet rich in whole grains, fruits, vegetables, and sufficient hydration promotes regular bowel movements and digestive comfort.

Consulting healthcare professionals and registered dietitians is paramount. These experts offer personalized guidance, tailoring dietary recommendations to an individual's specific needs and the severity of their condition. With their support, individuals can navigate the complexities of diverticulitis, making informed choices that promote intestinal health and overall well-being.

In essence, the proper diet, coupled with medical advice, empowers individuals to take control of their diverticulitis. By fostering a symbiotic relationship between mindful nutrition and professional guidance, managing diverticulitis becomes not just a challenge met but a hurdle overcome, enabling a life of comfort and vitality.

www.ingramcontent.com/pod-product-compliance
Lightning Source LLC
Chambersburg PA
CBHW050738260726

48661CB00001B/295

9798887062191 3